ROSACEA

Revealed: Understanding Rosacea and Developing Powerful Skin Care Techniques, Treatments, and Strategies

CHAD BRUNO

Table of Contents

Introductory

Redness, broken blood vessels, and, in certain circumstances, the appearance of tiny, pus-filled bumps or pimples can all be symptoms of rosacea, a chronic skin disorder that mostly affects the face. It frequently begins with a propensity to blush or flush more easily than other people and can evolve to a more persistent and extensive redness of the face. Dry, scratchy, and sometimes thicker skin on the nose (a disease called rhinophyma) are other frequent rosacea symptoms.

• Although the precise etiology of rosacea is unknown, it is thought to include interactions between genes, the environment, and blood vessels. Exposure to sunshine, hot or spicy foods, alcohol, stress, and even some skincare products can all bring on an episode of rosacea for some people.

• Medical treatment, lifestyle modifications, and proper skin care all have a role in reducing the severity of rosacea and keeping it under control. In order to find the best treatment for their unique symptoms, people with rosacea should consult a dermatologist.

Medication (including oral and topical), laser therapy, and avoiding triggers through lifestyle changes are common treatments.

Despite the fact that rosacea is a long-term skin condition, it is treatable and, with the right care, the symptoms and discomfort it causes can be greatly reduced. Consult a medical expert for a proper diagnosis and treatment plan if you experience rosacea symptoms like red, irritated skin or think you might have rosacea.

CHAPTER ONE
Rosacea Subtypes and Types

Rosacea is a multifaceted skin disorder with a wide range of possible presentations. The National Rosacea Society presently distinguishes between four primary kinds of rosacea, which have developed throughout time:

1.Rosacea,

Erythematotelangiectatic (ETR):

• The central face remains red (erythema) and visible blood vessels (telangiectasia) in this subtype. Skin may feel sensitive, scorching, or stinging for those with ETR, and they may also flush easily.

2. Rosacea, Papulopustular

• In this kind, which is sometimes called "acne rosacea," the center face becomes red and swollen and develops papules (small, red bumps) and pustules (pimples with pus). It can be easily confused for acne.

3. Rosacea Phymatosa:

• Rhinophyma is the most common skin thickening caused by phymatous rosacea, however it can also occur on the chin, forehead, cheeks, and ears. The skin may expand and develop bumps in certain spots.

4. Eye-related Rosacea:

• The eyes and eyelids are the most commonly affected areas by ocular rosacea. Cysts on the eyelids are another symptom, along with redness, dryness, and irritation of the eyes. It may be uncomfortable or even affect your eyesight, and it's often linked to other forms of rosacea.

The complexity of rosacea is reflected in its many possible manifestations; in addition to the four basic categories, some patients may exhibit a combination of symptoms from many subtypes. It's necessary to visit a dermatologist for a proper diagnosis and tailored treatment plan, as treatments can differ depending on the specific subtype and severity of rosacea. An individual's quality of life may be improved by early diagnosis and treatment.

Reasons & Prompts

Although the precise etiology of rosacea is unknown, it is thought to include interactions between genes, the environment, and blood vessels. Although the actual etiology of rosacea might vary from person to person, there are a number of risk factors that have been linked to the condition's onset and worsening:

1. There is some indication that rosacea has a hereditary component and so may run in families. A increased chance of acquiring rosacea is associated with a family history of the disorder.

2. Abnormal Blood Vessels: Changes in blood vessels in the skin, leading to increased blood flow and the creation of visible blood vessels (telangiectasia), are believed to have a role in the development of rosacea.

3. Inflammation and redness in rosacea may be the result of an inappropriate reaction from the immune system.

4. Increased populations of demodex mites, which are tiny parasites that live on humans naturally, may have a role in the etiology of rosacea.

5. Certain environmental conditions and triggers might bring out the worst in your rosacea. Common precipitants consist of:

• **Sunlight:** People with fair skin are more likely to experience an increase in redness and flare-ups when exposed to sunlight.

• **Hot Weather:** Rosacea flare-ups are often brought on by exposure to high temperatures and humidity.

Consuming spicy meals or beverages that are too hot might cause flushing and facial redness.

- **Alcohol:** Alcoholic beverages, especially red wine and some hard liquors, can provoke flushing and aggravate rosacea symptoms.

Tea, coffee, and other hot liquids may make symptoms worse.

Causes of flushes and flare-ups include emotional tension or worry.

Skincare products that are too harsh or irritating, especially those that contain alcohol or perfumes, might exacerbate rosacea.

Medication: o Rosacea can be triggered or made worse by some drugs. These include vasodilators and topical steroids.

It's worth noting that the causes of rosacea might differ from person to person. Managing the illness requires awareness of and avoidance of the factors that set off symptoms for the individual. Modifying one's lifestyle, using topical or oral drugs, and, in rare situations, undergoing laser or light therapy are all part of the standard protocol for treating this skin condition. If you suspect you have rosacea or are experiencing symptoms, check with a dermatologist for an accurate diagnosis and personalized treatment suggestions.

CHAPTER TWO
Symptoms and Indicators

Rosacea can present itself in a variety of ways, and the severity of its symptoms can vary from person to person. The most common rosacea symptoms are:

1. Facial Redness (Erythema): Persistent redness, particularly in the middle face, is a feature of rosacea. This flushing of the skin may be intermittent or more persistent.

2. Small, broken blood vessels on the skin's surface (also known as telangiectasia) can create a spiderweb or web-like pattern on the skin.

3. The face of a person with rosacea may turn red suddenly and temporarily due to a reaction to heat, sunshine, stress, or even particular meals and beverages.

4. Some people with rosacea experience the development of red, solid bumps known as papules, and pus-filled pimples known as pustules. Sometimes misdiagnosed as acne, this kind of rosacea is known as papulopustular rosacea.

5. Sensations of burning or stinging are common complaints from those who suffer with rosacea.

6. Skin that is dry or irritated often has a tight, dry, and irritated feel and may even appear scaly.

7. The skin on the nose (rhinophyma) and other parts of the face might thicken and become bumpy in more severe cases of rosacea, especially in men.

8. The eyes can be affected by ocular rosacea, resulting in redness, dryness, irritation, and even cysts on the eyelids.

9. Facial edema, especially in the area surrounding the nose, is another possible sign.

10.Some people with rosacea may have sensitive skin that has an adverse reaction to skincare products, resulting in heightened redness and irritation.

Some people with rosacea may not experience any of these symptoms at all. Some people with rosacea may have mild symptoms like redness and flushing, while others may experience more severe symptoms including papules, pustules, and thickened skin. A dermatologist or other medical professional can diagnose rosacea and provide guidance on how best to treat the condition and its symptoms. To manage the illness and lessen its effects on the skin, early identification and treatment is essential.

Classification and Diagnosis

Typically, a dermatologist or other healthcare physician with experience in skin disorders will diagnose and classify rosacea. Clinical examination, medical history evaluation, and extra testing to rule out other illnesses that may present similarly to rosacea all contribute to the diagnosis. Here are the procedures for identifying and categorizing rosacea:

• In a clinical examination, the doctor will look at the patient's face and skin to see whether there are any obvious symptoms. Examining the skin involves looking for signs of inflammation such as redness, visible blood vessels (telangiectasia), papules, pustules, and thickness.

• The patient's medical history will be discussed with the doctor, who will inquire about the patient's rosacea diagnosis, previous skin disorders, and current symptoms. Sunlight, hot and spicy foods, alcohol, and certain skincare practices will all be mentioned as potential irritants.

• Care providers may use differential diagnosis to rule out less serious skin disorders that produce similar symptoms. Conditions include acne, lupus, seborrheic dermatitis, and contact dermatitis may have overlapping features with rosacea. Therefore, it is crucial to tell rosacea apart from these other illnesses.

• The subtype of rosacea will be determined when the doctor examines the patient and makes a determination based on the patient's reported symptoms. Erythematotelangiectatic rosacea (ETR), papulopustular rosacea, phymatous rosacea, and ocular rosacea are the four primary subtypes of rosacea. It's possible that some people exhibit characteristics of multiple categories.

• Medical professionals may also assign a severity rating to the patient's rosacea, which may vary from mild to severe. This evaluation is used to direct further care.

• After a diagnosis has been made along with a determination of the condition's subtype and severity, the patient will get information about the disease, its causes, and potential therapies from the treating physician. Lifestyle adjustments and skincare treatments to manage rosacea may also be discussed.

• **Plan of Care:** A unique treatment strategy is created after a thorough evaluation and diagnosis. Topical and/or oral drugs, laser or light therapy, and suggested skin care routines may all be a part of this strategy.

If you think you have rosacea, consult a doctor right away; don't try to diagnose it on your own or cure it yourself. The disorder can be managed, its effects lessened, and the patient's quality of life enhanced with prompt diagnosis and treatment.

CHAPTER THREE
Recognizing and Avoiding Precipitating Factors

One of the most important aspects of rosacea management is recognizing and avoiding triggers. By detecting and limiting the things that increase your rosacea symptoms, you can help lessen redness, flushing, and associated discomfort. Here are some typical causes of anxiety and advice for avoiding them:

1. Start by documenting your routine, including what you eat and drink, what you use for skincare, and how your skin looks and feels.

Take note of the times that your rosacea symptoms worsen. You may be able to recognize patterns and understand causes as time goes on.

2. Every day, even on cloudy days, you should put on sunscreen with a high SPF and broad-spectrum protection to protect yourself from the sun. Sunglasses and a hat with a wide brim are essential outdoor accessories. Seek shelter and limit sun exposure during peak hours.

3. When temperatures soar, it's important to remember to keep your cool. If you can, stay out of the heat and humidity by using fans or air conditioning.

4. Reduce or eliminate your intake of spicy foods if you find that they aggravate your rosacea. Go with the gentler options.

5. Limit or avoid alcohol consumption if you notice that it exacerbates your symptoms. Wine, especially red wine, can be an allergen for some people.

6. If drinking hot liquids, such as coffee or tea, makes your symptoms worse, try waiting until they cool down a bit before drinking them.

You may try ordering iced versions of your usual drinks.

7. Flare-ups can be mitigated by practicing stress management strategies including yoga, meditation, deep breathing exercises, or engaging in regular physical activity.

8. Products for the Skin Be kind to your skin by using mild, fragrance-free products made specifically for sensitive skin types. Stay away from anything that contains alcohol, menthol, or anything else that can cause irritation. Perform patch testing on new goods to verify they don't increase your symptoms.

9. Rosacea can be made worse by exposure to environmental factors like as wind and extreme cold. If you live in an area where the air is often dry, a humidifier can help.

10. Medication: Some drugs can bring on or aggravate rosacea. Flare-ups could be the result of a medicine you're taking, so it's important to talk to your doctor about possible alternatives.

11. Rosacea can be triggered by overheating, so it's best to avoid activities like vigorous exercise, hot baths, and saunas. Choose tepid activities and soaks.

12. Diet: Certain foods and drinks, such as spicy foods and alcohol, might be triggers for some people. It's crucial to recognize and avoid these individual causes of distress.

13. Triggers can be very specific to an individual, so keep that in mind. What aggravates rosacea in one person might have no effect on another. Pay attention to your body's responses and modify your trigger avoidance accordingly.

When you know what sets off your rosacea flare-ups, you can take steps to prevent them. This, in addition to the medical treatment your doctor has given, can help you control your rosacea and bring relief to your skin. In order to come up with a good management plan, it is crucial to collaborate closely with a dermatologist or other healthcare professional.

Influences from both genes and the environment

Genetic and environmental factors both play a role in the development of rosacea. In order to effectively manage rosacea, it can be helpful to gain insight into the role that these factors have in its onset and progression.

Factors of Heredity:

1. Evidence suggests a genetic susceptibility plays a role in rosacea, and a family history of the condition is one possible indicator. A increased chance of acquiring rosacea is associated with a family history of the disorder. The greater prevalence of rosacea within families suggests a genetic relationship, but the precise genes involved have yet to be found.

2. Rosacea appears to be more prevalent in some ethnic groups than others. Fair-skinned individuals, especially those of Celtic or Northern European origin, are at a higher risk. Rosacea, however, affects people of all racial and cultural backgrounds equally.

3. Certain genetic variants have been linked to increased risk of developing rosacea, according to studies. These variations have been shown to influence vascular and immune system function, two key areas in the pathogenesis of rosacea.

• Sunlight and ultraviolet (UV) radiation are a prominent cause of rosacea flare-ups. Sunlight causes skin irritation and can cause blood vessels to enlarge. Sunscreen and other sun protection measures are crucial for rosacea sufferers.

• Hot and humid conditions can aggravate rosacea symptoms and trigger flushing. Problems can also arise from the presence of cold and windy weather. Keeping the house at a steady temperature is one way to lessen the impact of these external factors.

• **Diet:** Spicy meals and alcohol are known to cause flushing and redness in persons with rosacea. It may be helpful to learn to recognize and avoid these food triggers.

• Rosacea symptoms may be made worse by emotional stress. Reducing stress-related episodes may be possible with the use of stress management strategies including yoga, meditation, and therapy.

• **Skincare Products**: Skincare products that are too harsh and contain alcohol, perfumes, or other irritants can make rosacea worse. Select hypoallergenic, mild, and soothing skin care products.

• Medications, particularly topical steroid creams and vasodilators, have been linked to either the onset of rosacea or its exacerbation. Talk to your doctor about potential substitutions if you feel that a medicine is triggering your problems.

• The microorganisms that normally reside on the skin, such as Demodex mites, may have a role in rosacea. Both changes in the skin's microbiome and an increase in the mite population have been investigated as possible causes of eczema.

• **Hormonal Factors:** Hormonal variations may influence rosacea symptoms, particularly in women. Hormonal changes, such as those brought on by menopause or the use of hormonal birth control, can have an effect on rosacea.

We still don't fully understand the complicated interplay between genetic and environmental variables in rosacea. Some people may be genetically predisposed to developing rosacea, but environmental variables and triggers play a key influence in determining the onset and severity of symptoms. In order to properly manage rosacea and enhance the appearance and comfort of one's skin, it is recommended that one work with a dermatologist to develop a thorough management plan that takes into consideration both genetic and environmental factors.

CHAPTER FOUR
Rosacea Controlling

Rosacea is often treated with a combination of lifestyle adjustments, skin care, and medication. Key approaches to controlling rosacea include:

• You should see a dermatologist if you have been diagnosed with rosacea or if you think you might have it. They will be able to determine the precise nature of your rosacea, categorize its degree of severity, and advise you on the best course of therapy.

• Focus on figuring out what sets off your anxiety and then working to eliminate that trigger. Exposure to direct sunshine, extreme heat, spicy meals, alcohol, stress, and irritative skincare products are common causes of flare-ups.

• Wearing a wide-brimmed hat, sunglasses, and a high SPF broad-spectrum sunscreen every day, even on cloudy days, will help prevent sun damage to your skin. Seek shelter and limit sun exposure during peak hours.

• Use fragrance-free, mild skin care products made specifically for sensitive skin. Avoid products with alcohol, menthol, or other irritants. Perform patch testing on new goods to verify they don't increase your symptoms.

• Redness and inflammation can be treated with topical drugs prescribed by your dermatologist. These medications include metronidazole, azelaic acid, and brimonidine. Use these drugs exactly as prescribed.

• **Oral Medications:** In more severe situations, oral antibiotics like doxycycline or isotretinoin may be administered to manage inflammation and papules/pustules. Always listen to your doctor's advice when taking medication.

•	Visible blood vessels (telangiectasia) may respond well to laser therapy or other forms of light treatment. These blood arteries can be targeted and shrunk with laser treatments like intense pulsed light (IPL).

•	Eye care specialists (ophthalmologists) should be consulted for treatment of ocular rosacea. Treatment options may include eye drops and other therapies.

• To assist control stress-related episodes, try frequent physical activity, yoga, meditation, deep breathing exercises, or any combination of these.

• **Dietary Changes:** Determine which foods and drinks, such spicy meals and alcohol, aggravate your rosacea, and cut them out of your diet entirely. Keeping to a good diet plan might help with skin health in general.

• Maintaining a Comfortable Body Temperature is Essential, Especially in Hot Weather. Humidifiers, air conditioners, and fans should be used as required.

• Support groups for people with rosacea are a great way to get advice and encouragement from people who are also dealing with the condition.

• Maintain touch with your dermatologist for routine checkups and to discuss making any necessary alterations to your treatment plan.

• Make up for redness concealment should be hypoallergenic and formulated for sensitive skin. Makeup should never be scrubbed off the face; instead, use a soft cotton pad.

Keep in mind that treating rosacea is a gradual process, and that the methods that work for one individual may not be appropriate for another. Finding the right combination of treatments for your unique set of symptoms and triggers may require some experimentation. The best way to control rosacea is to be consistent and patient. To get the best outcomes from your therapy, you and your doctor should work together to create a tailor-made strategy.

Nutritional Diet

Some people get relief from their rosacea symptoms by making changes to their diet and nutrition. While there is no one-size-fits-all diet for rosacea, making specific dietary alterations and paying attention to potential triggers can help minimize the frequency and severity of flare-ups. Here are some suggestions for controlling rosacea through diet:

1. Recognize Trigger Foods Some people's rosacea symptoms might be triggered by eating or drinking certain things. Spicy foods, hot drinks, and alcohol are common dietary triggers. In order to determine which foods are aggravating your condition, you should keep a food diary.

2. Many people who suffer from rosacea are triggered by spicy foods because of capsaicin, the component responsible for the spiciness of peppers. Foods that are highly spiced with chili peppers and other hot spices should be limited or avoided.

3. Red wine, in particular, is known to bring on flushing and redness in certain people with rosacea. If drinking alcohol exacerbates your symptoms, you may want to cut back or switch to something less likely to do so.

4. Cool and Hydrating Foods: Incorporate foods that have a cooling and hydrating effect on the body. Examples of foods that may help alleviate facial redness and heat sensations include cucumbers, watermelon, and mint.

5. Antioxidant-Rich Meals: Antioxidant-rich meals can enhance general skin health. Fruits and vegetables are excellent sources of anti-oxidants, vitamins, and minerals, so be sure to eat plenty of them. Fruits, vegetables, and citrus are all great options.

6. Fatty fish (salmon, mackerel, sardines), flaxseeds, and walnuts are high in omega-3 fatty acids and may help reduce rosacea-related redness and inflammation due to their anti-inflammatory effects.

7. Keeping yourself adequately hydrated is crucial to the upkeep of your skin's health. Maintaining hydrated skin requires regular use of water.

8. Dietary Balance: Aim for a diet that provides a wide range of nutrients. In order to reduce inflammation, you should limit your intake of processed and sugary foods.

9. Allergic reactions or sensitivities to certain foods may have a role in the development of rosacea in certain people. Consider getting tested for food allergies or talking to a doctor if you have reason to believe that a particular food is the source of your health problems.

10. Supplements: Talk to your doctor before taking any vitamins or minerals, as they can advise you on whether or not taking things like niacinamide, zinc, or vitamin C would help your condition.

Keep in mind that rosacea sufferers can have wildly varying responses to food factors. Not everyone will benefit from the same strategies. In order to discover the best dietary changes for your unique illness and symptoms, it is important to engage closely with a healthcare expert, in this case a dermatologist. A doctor can also help you determine if your diet is causing or aggravating your rosacea.

CHAPTER FIVE
How to Manage Rosacea

Rosacea is a frustrating ailment to live with because it not only alters your appearance but also causes pain and embarrassment. However, rosacea can be controlled and the quality of life enhanced with the help of the correct methods and people. Some strategies for managing rosacea are outlined below.

• Consult a Dermatologist or Healthcare Provider. This is the first step in dealing with rosacea. They are qualified to identify your specific kind of rosacea and provide you with tailored recommendations for relieving your symptoms.

• Take the time to educate yourself on rosacea. Feeling more in charge of the situation is possible after learning about the ailment, its causes, and the options for therapy.

• Be True to Your therapy Plan: Stick to the course of therapy that has been established between you and your doctor. Topical or oral drugs, changes in diet and exercise, and special skin care routines are all possibilities.

• **Controlling Triggers:** Recognizing and avoiding the things those bring on flare-ups of rosacea. Maintaining a journal detailing stressful events can be beneficial.

• Skincare Products for Sensitive Skin Should Be Mild Use products that are mild and fragrance-free. Don't use anything that contains alcohol or other skin irritants. Find out what your dermatologist recommends by talking to them.

• Protect your skin from the sun by seeking out shade, wearing protective clothing, sunglasses, and using sunscreen.

• Manage your stress by engaging in stress-reduction activities, such as yoga, meditation, or deep breathing exercises.

• Keep your skin hydrated and your skin health in check by drinking plenty of water.

• Join a local rosacea support group or find a comparable online community to share your experiences with others. It might be reassuring to share your opinions and learn from those of others.

• When applying cosmetics or caring for your skin, choose products that are hypoallergenic and mild. Makeup with a greenish tinge helps hide facial redness.

Makeup should never be scrubbed off, but instead removed carefully.

• If you suspect you have ocular rosacea, it is highly recommended that you schedule an appointment with an ophthalmologist right away.

• Be an advocate for yourself by being upfront about your health with loved ones and coworkers. Educate them about rosacea to reduce misunderstandings and myths.

• Emotional support is helpful for those suffering from rosacea. You should think about getting help from a mental health expert if your rosacea has caused you to feel depressed, anxious, or low in self-esteem.

• Remind yourself that your rosacea is not who you are. Focus on your traits, talents, and hobbies that make you distinct and confident. Have faith in yourself; it will help you get through this.

• Follow up with your dermatologist on a regular basis for exams and to make any necessary adjustments to your therapy.

When treating rosacea, patience and persistence are key. There may not be a cure for rosacea, but with the right treatment, most people can significantly improve their skin's appearance and comfort. The best way to deal with rosacea is to surround yourself with positive people, educate yourself, and take care of your mental health.

Regular Skin Care

Even if you don't have a skin disease like rosacea, a regular skincare routine can help keep your skin healthy and comfortable. The following is a general guideline for skin care that can be modified to meet your own needs and preferences:

Get Ready for the Day:

• Use a cleanser that is hypoallergenic and formulated for dry skin. If you suffer from rosacea, it's best to steer clear of abrasive cleansers.

• Choose an alcohol-free toner that is hypoallergenic if you have sensitive skin, if you decide to use a toner. Applying a toner helps maintain a healthy skin pH.

• Treatment (If Prescribed): Apply any topical drugs or therapies suggested by your dermatologist.

• To avoid dryness and keep your skin hydrated, use a noncomedogenic, fragrance-free moisturizer. Try to find anything that will protect you from the harmful effects of your surroundings.

• **Sunscreen:** Apply a broad-spectrum, SPF 30 or higher sunscreen. Sun protection is crucial, as sun exposure can trigger rosacea symptoms.

The Nightly Ritual:

• Makeup, debris, and pollutants may all be easily washed away with the same mild cleanser you use first thing in the morning. If you put on sunscreen or cosmetics, you might need to wash your face twice.

• Apply a toner if you like, just like you did in the morning.

• Apply any topical drugs or therapies recommended by your doctor.

4. To keep your skin supple and happy, apply a moisturizer of your choice.

• When it comes to exfoliation, delicate skin should be protected from strong physical exfoliants like scrubs. Under a dermatologist's supervision, a chemical exfoliator (alpha hydroxy acids or beta hydroxy acids) is a good option for those who want to exfoliate.

• **Cosmetics:** If you have sensitive skin or rosacea, go for cosmetics made for certain skin types. Makeup with a greenish tinge helps hide facial redness. Makeup should be removed carefully to prevent skin irritation.

• Perform a patch test to see if there are any allergic reactions before using a new skin care product.

• Applying a cool, moist cloth to your face might help soothe inflamed or irritated skin.

• The health of your skin can be affected by your lifestyle choices, so it's important to eat well, drink plenty of water, and deal with stress well.

• **Avoid Triggers:** Identify and avoid your unique rosacea triggers, such as certain foods, environmental conditions, and stress.

Choose moderate, non-irritating products and stick to your routine for the best results when caring for rosacea-prone skin. Also, before making any major adjustments to your skincare routine, it's smart to check in with your dermatologist for recommendations on effective products to use. They'll be able to provide you advice that works for your subtype and skin condition.

One kind of rosacea, known as ocular rosacea, manifests particularly in the eye area. It's possible to have this skin condition alone or in tandem with other rosacea varieties. Recognizing and effectively treating ocular rosacea is essential for alleviating the associated discomfort and symptoms. **Some important points about ocular rosacea are as follows:**

Ocular rosacea symptoms include:

• Ocular rosacea is characterized by red or bloodshot eyes.

• Ocular rosacea is commonly associated with dry, inflamed eyes.

• Ocular rosacea sufferers often report a burning or stinging feeling in their eyes.

• The eyes may feel gritty, as if a foreign object were lodged inside them.

• crying: In an ironic twist, ocular rosacea can cause excessive crying as the eyes try to compensate for dryness.

• Light Sensitivity (Photophobia): People with ocular rosacea may have a heightened sensitivity to light.

• Inflammation of the Eyelids: Blepharitis and Chalazia are cysts that can form on the eyelids as a result of this illness.

Ocular rosacea treatment:

Combining medical therapy with behavioral modifications is the usual approach to controlling ocular rosacea. Some typical methods are as follows:

• Closing your eyes and applying a warm compress might help alleviate symptoms and promote better eyelid hygiene. This can alleviate the pain and unclog the tear ducts' oil glands.

• Use of a mild cleanser or lid wipes on a regular basis, as prescribed by your eye doctor, can aid in the control of blepharitis and the avoidance of problems.

• Over-the-counter lubricating eye drops (sometimes known as "artificial tears") can help relieve dryness and other symptoms, such as gritty or burning eyes.

• In some circumstances, a doctor may recommend using medicated eye drops or ointments to reduce the swelling and redness.

• Antibiotics like tetracycline and doxycycline, taken orally, may be prescribed by your doctor to reduce inflammation and manage ocular rosacea.

• **Environmental Control:** Avoiding triggers including sunlight, wind, and dust can help prevent eye irritation. Sunglasses with ultraviolet (UV) protection are also recommended.

• It is recommended that you see an ophthalmologist or other eye doctor who specializes in the treatment of ocular rosacea. They are qualified to offer specialist assistance and advice.

• Maintain consistent contact with your eye doctor so that your ocular rosacea can be treated and monitored effectively.

Ocular rosacea can be a persistent problem that needs ongoing treatment. Maintaining good eye health and avoiding problems requires prompt diagnosis and prompt treatment. Warning signs of ocular rosacea should trigger a visit to the doctor for a proper diagnosis and treatment plan.

A good perspective and effective coping mechanisms make it possible to lead a satisfying life despite rosacea. Although rosacea can be persistent, it is treatable, and many people with the illness enjoy normal, productive lives. Some advice on how to manage life with rosacea:

• Seek the Advice of Dermatologist
First things first, get the advice of a dermatologist. They will be able to identify the specific form of rosacea

you have and prescribe a treatment regimen tailored specifically to your needs.

• Adhere to the treatment plan prescribed by your dermatologist, which may include of topical or oral drugs, changes to your lifestyle, and/or skin care regimens.

• **Skincare Routine:** Create a routine that is gentle on your skin by utilizing hypoallergenic, fragrance-free products made for sensitive skin. Don't use anything too abrasive on your skin.

• Use a broad-spectrum sunscreen, protective clothes, sunglasses, and shade to keep UV rays from causing skin irritation.

• Manage your rosacea by avoiding the things that bring on flare-ups for you individually (known as "triggers"). Keep a diary detailing the instances that triggered you.

• Makeup and skin care products should be chosen with the user's sensitive skin in mind. Makeup with a greenish tinge helps hide facial redness. Always be careful when removing makeup.

• Reduce stressful episodes by practicing relaxation methods like yoga, meditation, deep breathing exercises, or frequent physical activity.

• **Stay Hydrated:** Ensure you drink enough water to maintain skin hydration and overall well-being.

• Care for your eyes as recommended by your ophthalmologist if you have ocular rosacea.

• Adopt a diet high in anti-oxidant-rich fruits, vegetables, and whole grains to promote radiant skin. Determine and control any dietary factors that may be contributing to your condition.

• Join a rosacea support group or a community online where you can talk to other people who understand what it's like to live with the condition and offer and receive encouragement.

• Help dispel myths and misconceptions about rosacea by sharing your knowledge with friends, family, and coworkers.

• Focus on your strengths, hobbies, and other aspects of yourself that you know inspire confidence. Keep in mind that rosacea is not who you are.

• In the event that rosacea-related emotional distress, sadness, or anxiety persists despite treatment, professional mental health assistance should be sought.

• **Regular Follow-Ups:** Stay in contact with your dermatologist for regular check-ups and modifications to your treatment plan.

• Use common sense measures, such as applying warm compresses or adjusting the temperature and humidity in the room, to alleviate the symptoms.

• Self-Advocacy as a Patient Do what you can to get others to understand and help you by being upfront about your condition and your needs.

Maintaining a high quality of life while dealing with rosacea necessitates diligent attention to self-care, education, and, when necessary, professional assistance. You can control rosacea, lessen its impact on your life, and live the way you want to if you have the correct treatment plan and a strong social support system.

Conclusion

rosacea is a chronic skin ailment that usually affects the face and, in rare circumstances, the eyes. Redness, broken capillaries, papules, pustules, and thicker skin are only few of the possible outward signs. Rosacea is influenced by both hereditary and environmental factors, and avoiding triggers is a common treatment strategy.

• A dermatologist is needed to properly diagnose and categorize rosacea, as each patient has a unique treatment approach based on their specific subtype and severity level. Topical and oral drugs, lifestyle adjustments, skincare routines, and laser or light therapy are all viable options for management. Specialized eye care and therapy are necessary for the subtype of rosacea known as ocular rosacea.

Learning about rosacea, getting medical advice, sticking to a tailored treatment plan, and making adjustments to one's lifestyle can all assist. Living well with rosacea requires a combination of medical treatment, self-care, and social support.

Individuals with rosacea can effectively manage their illness, reduce discomfort, and have a good quality of life by following the recommendations of healthcare specialists, implementing practical solutions, and keeping a healthy lifestyle.

THE END

www.ingramcontent.com/pod-product-compliance
Lightning Source LLC
Chambersburg PA
CBHW070031260726
48658CB00002B/584